THE CURE FOR MENTAL ILLNESS

Cover illustration by Randy Sawmiller.

Printed in the United States of America

First Printing, 2025

ISBN 979-8-89390-004-0

Library of Congress Control Number: Pending
Ordering Information: Special discounts are available on quantity purchases by bookstores, corporations, associations, and others. For details, contact the publisher at sales@braughlerbooks.com or at 937-58-BOOKS.

For questions or comments about this book, please write to info@braughlerbooks.com.

Braughler™ Books
braughlerbooks.com

THE CURE FOR MENTAL ILLNESS

KRISTINE GORDON

Table of Contents

Introduction

Healing does not follow drugs or hocus pocus. Healing is a total investment by the healer to the healee, and the healee to health. It is love.

Please allow me to introduce myself. I am a psychotherapist, professor, and designer of unique programs for mental health. I have written articles that reached a worldwide audience and gave a plenary speech to an international audience of 1,000-plus mental health professionals and non-professionals. I also put together a workshop for "unprofessionals," resulting in the accolades of some and the wrath of others. Why, I asked myself, didn't they want to hear the truth? Why aren't they relieved that such a "professional" is speaking the truth? As Jack Nicholson once said, they "can't handle the truth." So true, so true.

Several years ago, I was given Bactrim, which is an antibiotic. I had an allergic reaction to the Bactrim, and, with no warning, I went into a coma. The coma landed me on life support, and the doctors gave me a 2% chance to live. I had a near-death experience just prior to emerging from that coma. Interestingly, none of the doctors would tell me what happened that put me in a coma until an outspoken doctor I met in rehab told me the truth. I mention this, as this captures the ambiance of current-day psychiatry.

While I was in this coma, I saw my mother, father, and grandmother, who were all long gone. It was not a dream. It was reality. We communicated with love, not with words. I was so very, very happy to see them after such a long time. Suddenly, they sent the message that I needed to leave them quickly. I turned and ran. I ran as fast as I had as a child and was out of breath. I stopped. In front of me were my son and daughter. Again, no words were said, just love. I hugged them with all my being. I woke up to a nurse saying, "Welcome back!"

This led me to question the meaning of my life. Questions I had not asked since my undergraduate days studying psychology and philosophy. Why am I here? Questions I did not have the time or energy to ask for many years. As a single parent, I was a gerbil on a wheel, keeping body and soul together. What am I doing here?

The immediate outcome, of course, was evident in the near-death experience. I am here to care for my children. It is my first and last priority. I kept questioning, asking, thinking that there must be something else. Something I was missing. "What is it? What is it?" I repeated again and again. The answer, as often is the case, was right in front of me. I needed to get the honest, unadulterated truth out about the practices in the mental health field. The odds are against me as I watch "expert" after "expert" in the media parlaying their answers. Believe what you choose. I am speaking the truth. My job is only to enlighten you and not to convert you if you are a believer in cognitive, trauma, medication, or whatever type of therapy. I have learned that I have never changed anyone; they have changed themselves.

I currently work as a therapist at your local, neighborhood mental health clinic. Trust me, I use the term health very loosely. Most of the time, these centers are promoting mental dysfunction and drug dependence, not mental well-being. I wrestle daily with the debate of whether I am promoting dysfunction or am a beacon of light in a dark and dreary place. I, of course, prefer the latter. I know there are times due to battle fatigue, I too have promoted dysfunction.

Chapter 1:

The Club and All You Need Is Love

The mental health "system," which is more of a helter-skelter hodgepodge of stuff, will focus on your symptoms and not on your dreams.

Prior to my awakening regarding mental health—or, as it was called at the time, mental illness—I was a believer. I diligently studied Piaget, Skinner, all the philosophers, etc. etc. looking for the answer. There were tidbits of reality in each approach. If you repeatedly give a kid a cookie when he or she does something good, chances are that the kid will repeat the desired behavior. Unfortunately, the world doesn't always dole out cookies. Keep in mind, the beginning of psychology was philosophy—men in togas who were wealthy enough to sit around and observe the action and write their comments. Do we have philosophers today? Of course. And now, we call them psychologists. Psychology, for the most part, has the equivalent scientific basis as philosophy—that being little to none.

I went from job to job in hopes of finding "the answer." I found bureaucracies that allowed for superficial relationships but supplied other things, such as college tuition if you could maneuver the person into and around the bureaucracy. I found low-paying jobs in residential programs located in what was labeled the "psychiatric ghetto." It was always a "residential program" instead of the home people wanted and needed. I taught folks meditation long before it was the newest fad and a movement in the field. It was an anti-anxiety, depression-lifting, focusing vehicle long before—and less addictive and deadly than—Adderall, Librium, etc. Later, the insurance companies would agree, since teaching meditation is far less costly than paying for the drugs. This did, however, create a conflict with the pharmaceutical companies, which, in response, created a multitude of additional antidepressants for your psychic pleasure. The problem is that generally, they don't work and don't even provide the high you can get from Clonidine, Adderall, etc.

I will not bore you with the details of the plethora of work situations I experienced. I did a post-graduate degree fellowship, one of five awarded statewide called "Arts and Human Services." I did enjoy that and nearly sent many bureaucrats into cardiac arrest when I had mentally ill folks working in stained glass. They admitted that the works we did were quite beautiful but said that they must be anti-therapeutic, because the only thing that crazy people do with broken glass, they claimed, is to slit their wrists. Ah, stigma at its finest.

Somehow, I moved ahead and became an "expert," and with the assistance of a friend, was recruited to set up programs at our local state hospital. This was the period of deinstitutionalization. Translated, this meant that they discovered that it was cheaper to get people out of the state hospitals and back into the communities. Keep in mind that when the state hospitals began, they were lauded as the answer to folks challenged by anxiety, depression, hallucinations, or whatever symptoms they were experiencing. It also met the needs of disgruntled husbands who wanted to jettison their current wife and such. The strange phenomenon was that in the process of getting people into the community, a large amount of the state money evaporated into thin air! This was perhaps the opposite of a miracle for those needing it, but not for those orchestrating the process.

I recall my first day as the director of vocational rehabilitation at Worcester State Hospital. I was given a key ring the size of one any guard at any penitentiary might have. There were usually a set of two locked doors to keep the prisoners—oops, patients—in and others out.

I recall the first time unlocking the first door and entering, and then the door SLAMMING behind me. Slamming is not an adequate description. As the gust of wind it created pushed me down the short corridor to the next door, I frantically searched the key ring for the key to that door. I made a bargain with God that I would never break the law or become crazy and end up in the state hospital or penitentiary. I could only imagine what this might feel like if you did not have a set of keys in your hand. There were keys and burly guards or mental health/illness assistants to keep everyone in line. And they marveled at why people would get aggressive. I marveled at why this did not happen more frequently.

I did not last very long at Worcester State Hospital. I was tired of struggling with whether I was part of the problem or solving the problem. When it became clear that I was the problem, I left. I tried to fight the good fight but was greatly outnumbered. The Worcester State Hospital became The Recovery Center with little change except a new building. I had gone to a six-week training program while I worked at Mass. Rehab. Every state has a Mass. Rehab, as federal law mandates this to help folks with disabilities live independently and return to work.

I was exposed to Fountain House at that time and witnessed how people who had been thrown away via the state hospital system were coming back to life. There was an opening at a fledgling club near me. I applied and was dubbed "Social Director." Fun? Not so much. This was certainly no cruise ship.

I began my job full of hope and was eager to see the miracles at Fountain House transferred to a club near me. The director was an antisocial social worker. The links that could help people return to or begin their lives were tenuous at best, and the club ambiance was debilitating. I watched one day as the director imitated tap dancing and playing a violin while a member recounted the difficulties he was having at home. There must be respect. There must be caring. It is not only how a program is set up; it is also who is in charge. It is those moment-to-moment affirming interactions that will make or break you and the people you are working with. Onward to my next mission.

My next mission remains the most rewarding and honest experience of my career. I heard it through the grapevine that the city where I lived was starting a clubhouse. Well, I thought, it's got to work better than the last one. The roots of Fountain House tell you there was love in the beginning. The founders were two moms who were worried about their children who had been "deinstitutionalized" and were wandering the streets of New York City. The same concern started the Genesis Club. Parents of the deinstitutionalized kids—frequently young adults in Worcester, Massachusetts—wanted the same thing. They wanted their children to be all they could be despite mental illness. The neighborhood mental health centers for the most part provided a genre where the theme was debilitating participants. "God bless the child who's got his own" and those families who care whether their child has got his own.

"Free at last, free at last. Thank God almighty, we are free at last." Please excuse my use of expressions that perhaps have been overused. I do think they express better than I can the ambiance that existed when we started the club. I was hired as assistant director and soon after the club began, I was named program director. As is familiar to many women, I was doing the bulk of the work and creativity, while my male boss was doing the bulk of the showcasing and the taking credit. No matter. I could finally live the principles I found dear in my personal and professional life.

One of the missions of the club was to liberate the folks being held at the local state hospital and the other psychiatric units in the city. I returned to the Worcester State Hospital. This time I had no keys; I had something better. I had the club members or the folks who had lived the horrors at the state hospital and their selfless dedication to liberate those who had been left behind. Here, there was no meaningless diagnosis. Here, there was caring and concern, the cornerstone of recovery and life. The relationships were honest and loving with those who had lost this long ago. Here, there was Millie, whom I had come to teach about the clubhouse model and who taught me more than I would ever learn from years of school and "experts." She taught me what really cures those buffeted and degraded by the system.

I am not saying that there are no rays of hope wherever one seeks help. As always, the answer was so very simple: love and respect for those who need us and love and respect for the work to be done. The endless dog-and-pony shows, as well as the snake oil salesmen, continue their work to this day, promising miracles and delivering little to nothing. Current examples of "snake oil sales" are ketamine and LSD. We have been the LSD route before thank you and I am still piecing together the resulting train wrecks. Who wouldn't love ketamine? Also known as "special K" the party drug. It's hard to be depressed when you are high.

The first time I met Millie, she was hovering around the circle that had formed as we spoke of the miracles that can happen. Wisely, she was skeptical after years of being degraded by the system. We made eye contact. I saw a glimmer of a twinkle that I knew instantly would be easily reignited. She had been labeled bipolar, whatever that means. It means little to those who know the truth about the system, diagnosing, and the DSM (the bible of mental illness), and it means much to those who promote it. Millie and I chatted for a bit after the group had concluded. She did not readily commit to trying out the club. "Fool me once, shame on you. Fool me twice, shame on me." Millie was no fool.

One day, as we were hustling and bustling around the activity of the club, I looked up, and there stood Millie. I was honored that she would trust me enough to come to Genesis Club. How simple it is to truly care and walk a mile in someone else's moccasins. How many walls are built up by the providers and consumers of the system to prevent this. Separate but equal, sort of and not really.

She showed me that the "clients" have their own subculture, a code of secrecy and ethics not to be shared with "them." It is rather ironic that true healing will only happen when these walls come tumbling down. The providers foster an "us vs. them" atmosphere under the guise of liability, confidentiality, and insurance policies. Is it ever respectful to dissect a person's life in front of a crowd of disinterested participants, which is usually called a staff meeting? It is respectful to assemble only those the person wants present. Period. Run, do not walk when you hear one of these "raison d'etre" to give validity to the moat around the "professional castle." The inmates will smile and flatter the guards.

Millie became a regular. Every day, I watched her as she did the work of the club and became a mentor and sometimes disciplinarian to members testing the limits. She did the job of the staff often more adeptly and in a more caring way than the hired staff.

Then it happened. Millie called me from the guest house—a rented house where the colleagues now coming from all over the world would stay as they learned about Genesis. Millie was serving as hostess for these folks. We were beginning to know and understand each other. The trust that is the bedrock of any relationship was being built stone by stone. She called.

It was late in the afternoon, and I was doing my usual running around—the life of full-time worker and full-time single mom. Millie didn't say anything to raise an alarm. She was "just checking in from the guest house." But my mom's sixth sense kicked in. I assured her all was well and that I would just be dropping by to say hey. As previously mentioned, the relationship is the cornerstone of treatment and recovery. She said okay and hung up. I had an uneasy feeling as I drove to the guest house. The feeling did not come from clinical skills but from the depth of our developing trust in a relationship.

I walked into the house and called Millie, trying to figure out where she was. After a brief search, I heard her call out, "In here."

I walked into the kitchen, and there sat Millie at the kitchen table, with a quart of Jack Daniels and her pills lined up nicely in a row. I looked at the bottle, which was half empty, then at the line of pills and at Millie. My "clinical assessment" was, "But you don't even drink."

Millie responded, "Yeah, I know."

"How many pills have you taken?"

"I'm not sure."

"I'm calling the ambulance."

"Yeah, okay."

I was hoping they would get her to the ER quicker than I could. The paramedics soon arrived. I explained the situation.

They nodded in agreement and gathered up the pill bottles to take with them.

"I will meet you at the ER," I told her. I watched as they walked Millie to the ambulance, and then I quickly headed to my car.

In retrospect, I minimized the behavior I had come to know too well and to respond to too well. I was panicked on the inside, and the outside remained calm. I wanted to cry for my friend and client Millie but kept it under control. I mimicked the "stiff upper lip" my mom had schooled me in. It is a behavior I have emulated over and over in my life when something catastrophic has happened to someone I care about, be they friend, family, client, or whatever label they may be assigned.

And therein lies the golden key to effective "treatment" or to relationships or to life. You must care. You must care—not on a superficial level, but on a spiritual, real level. For all those clinicians, providers, psychotherapists, or whatever title you choose or are given, if this is not the case, find another line of work. To all the "programs" that provide a superficial "answer," close your doors. You are doing more harm than good, sort of. Keep the faith that within your debilitating walls, there still will be those who genuinely care.

I arrived at the hospital to find Millie being tended to by means of being made to drink charcoal to absorb the whiskey and pills. I sat by her side when the nurses had finished their work. I kept checking to see if she needed anything, to assure myself that she wasn't going to die on me and to assure her that I genuinely cared.

Eventually, she said in her direct Millie way, "I'm not going to do that again." Part of this was that she did not want to physically go through this again, part of it was not to cause me the pain that I tried to hide, and part of it was thoughts of her children. Millie was discharged a day or two later according to whatever was the dictate of the insurance company at the time.

The reality is that if someone is determined to kill themselves, they will. Everyone knows the magic words to get out of or into the hospital. I later watched as a friend was whisked away to the ER by her therapist as their 45 minutes were up. In an effort to avoid any lawsuit, the therapist had sent her to the ER. Caring? Not so much. Common? Yes, very much. The trick, of course, is to care enough to respond to the hints a person gives you, so they will not harm themselves.

We resumed our work. Millie and I worked together on behalf of all the folks coming to the club, and it resulted in personal and professional growth that both she and I had never dreamed of. It would never have happened in the "models" that had become so familiar to both of us. All you need is love, dedication, and hard work. Millie had plenty of all to give.

Unfortunately, the clubhouse model can be just as ineffective if not done with these components. Therefore, clubhouses under the auspices of mental health centers generally die a slow, ineffective death.

One of the areas where we began to see miracles happen was around work. At this time, the only dream people could have regarding work was to be put in what were called workshops. If you are thinking Santa's elves, they were a long, long way from this. This was what was offered to folks regardless of what their own dreams and accomplishments were. Picture being a young woman who has dropped out of medical school, and the only option you are given for meaningful employment is piece work earning a few cents per piece in a dilapidated workplace. Not even minimum wage. If you weren't depressed before, you would be now.

These places still exist. They are not the answer for most folks, but they can be for a very SMALL minority of people who are seriously challenged. A person who is severely autistic who has little ability to speak or reason may need something like this to be able to work. Work has great significance in our culture, so it is important to include everyone. Creativity can be used in terms of the work, making it meaningful for all.

Millie and I began the job search on behalf of the club. I thought my own job searches had been arduous. Well, that was a piece of cake compared to job hunting for the club members at Genesis. Why is that? you may ask. Stigma was and currently is very much alive in our culture. Those "crazy people" might become homicidal maniacs at any moment. This would be very bad for business, no matter what type of business it was.

Although killing people is a totally separate problem from mental health challenges, for simplicity's sake, we like to regard them as one and the same. Why? One of the promoters of this thinking was and is your friendly neighborhood attorney. It was very creative of the one who thought up this concept in order to win what, to that point, had been unwinnable. What at first blush looks like an act of humanity has done more damage than lobotomies and electroshock therapy. "Not guilty by reason of insanity" promotes stigma at its finest.

I have watched case after case where attorneys resort to this when there is no other way out, and it has cost those who struggle a price one cannot calculate. Presented as an act of compassion, it is nothing of the sort. Harming others has nothing to do with mental health symptoms. There is a percentage of folks mentally ill or not capable of harming others. One has nothing to do with the other. For those people who are struggling with mental health issues, the only violence they might have a higher rate of than "normal" people is that of harming themselves. But that is of no use in a court case.

So off we went from one "potential" employer to the next. There really was no potential with most of the employers I met. I pounded the pavement for literally years to give the folks I was working with a chance at work. A chance at life.

Then one day as I was driving by a place called Shaughnessy Company, I figured, what the heck, I'll run in and pitch my spiel. What can they say? "No"? No had become what I expected. I went into a warehouse type of building where they stored the cranes that the company rented.

I walked up to Jim Shaughnessy and gave my presentation. We gave 100% coverage for any position they would allow us to fill AND several tax benefits. That wasn't what sold Jim, and I doubt he even heard the "tax benefits" part. Jim later told me that he had a brother who struggled and was thinking that this might be a way to help him. Jim's brother had been sitting in isolation and depression for years. Jim said yes! I thought I was hallucinating and later sent a follow-up thank you note just to be certain the job offer was real. All you need is love and many worn-down pairs of high heels. Thank you, Jim. Thank you, Jesus. Thank you, Buddha. Thank you for caring.

After many, many rejections, Jim and Millie spurred me on with my eternal job hunt. The rejection of all the folks I was job-seeking on behalf of became quite personal. I went to UMass Medical School in Worcester, Massachusetts, and thought "Okay, there must be a Jim somewhere in this place." If not a Jim, perhaps some pressure from affirmative action.

Then I met Tony, a nice guy who assured me he would get at least one department head to assist with my mission. I dropped by to see Tony for about two years, checking in to see if he had found the Holy Grail of department heads. Somehow, I kept bothering Tony. Somehow, I thought he was still trying. Lo and behold, one sunny afternoon in April, Tony called and said, "I have someone, and I have set up a time for you to meet with them."

I said, "Great, and thank you," not realizing at that time that this would be a real challenge for me. My mom passed away after months of suffering with cancer. The appointment was the day after she died. I went to the appointment and brought my stiffest upper lip. My mom, Dot, would have approved. I met with the department head and sealed the deal. Thank you, Jesus. Thank you, Buddha. Thank you, Tony, and thank you, Dot. This was probably the best tribute to her. Hundreds of folks at the club have used these jobs to get back on track or to begin their journey in pursuit of their dreams. Amen.

Eventually, I secured, with a little help from my friends, many transitional employment slots to fill the needs of the folks at the club. Another problem with mental health programs and unfortunately regarding some things Fountain House had fallen into the trap of having "the answer" and anything not consistent with the answer becomes unequivocally the wrong answer.

Transitional employment, which was a wonderful invention, also had the phenomenon known as "shooting oneself in the foot." Transitional employment jobs were "owned by the club." That is, members could use them for three months to a year to get their bearings again. They were then expected to give the opportunity and job to another member. I challenged this, as is my nature, when folks would get into their TE job and want to stay. They wanted it to be their forever job.

I was "shooting myself in the foot", since this meant that I had to retrieve my high heels and hit the pavement again. "Oh no!" said the administrative director at the time, as I was deemed the program director, which just meant I did most of the work and most of the creating. I reminded him that our job was to help folks get on with their lives and pursue their dreams. It was hard to disagree with this and hard to disagree with the fact that I had been doing and would continue to do all the legwork. These TE jobs miraculously became what I called "supported employment," and eventually, everybody was happy—even Fountain House, who adopted my new and improved model.

Another area that was off limits to folks who had been labeled "mentally ill" was education. Folks were relegated to assembling widgets and getting their GEDs. Somehow, there had always been the confusion or stigma, shall we say, that folks with mental health issues were incapable of attending college successfully. Millie and I decided it was time to dispel that rumor. We had folks at the club who were nurses, in medical school, and lawyers. Psychiatric symptoms should not preclude going to college.

I was teaching at a local college when Millie decided to apply there. We walked through the application process together. She was not familiar with such things, so of course she had the normal reaction of becoming anxious. We were the perfect dynamic duo. I was on turf that I was very familiar with, but to Millie, this was uncharted territory. Very simple. No psychobabble needed or helpful. She was too anxious to go to class and take notes. I went with her and took notes until her panic attacks subsided into a dull roar and she said with pride and confidence that she could handle it alone. My mission was accomplished, and I had been fired from my job.

In the meantime, it was the late 1980s, Atlantic Union College was looking for people to try their "new and innovative approach" to learning or distance-learning. I snatched up the free computers they were offering. It was divine intervention for those too anxious, too depressed, or hallucinating too much to go into the classroom. Word on the street spread to Boston

University, and they gave money to the local community college. So began the first supported education program.

Millie completed all her courses and graduated with honors at the same time as her daughter. With her brand-new degree in human services, I hired Millie at the club to continue the work she had already been doing. It was the work she loved and excelled at, and now she would be paid for it. We went along as you do in life, thinking things would never change. Of course, they did, and I headed to another program to direct it, and Millie came with me. This club was under the auspices of your "friendly neighborhood mental health center."

Anne, the assistant director, appraised me of the outrage that had been going on for years. Money was being pocketed by the center, leaving the club with little to nothing. The club was housed in a garage, and any fundraising we did, the center took a cut. We blew the whistle. This resulted in all of us being fired, and the head of DMH, Connie Dotto, disappearing into the sunset. Other DMH bureaucrats were "relocated" around the state, just like the catholic priests had been after sexual abuse. The center eventually had to repay a large sum of money, but to my way of thinking, it was not large enough. This will give you a feel for the ambiance of mental health centers that continues to this day.

Millie and I welcomed my daughter, who is now twenty-five years old. Time flies when I think of my friend who taught me so much about mental health, caring, life, and what a good human being is like. She passed away not too long after my daughter Maggie was born. Millie was relatively young, and knowing what I know now, I cannot help but attribute this in large part to the powerful psychiatric meds she took religiously. She probably could have functioned just as well without them. At the time, stopping medication was sacrilege and would have resulted in being sectioned back into the hospital.

Since then, there have been many brave individuals who have come forward to challenge this thinking. The "cure," as we currently know it, is not about drugs and the many dog-and-pony shows. Our system in this country is driven by pharmaceuticals and by how we define mental illness by including psychiatry with other disciplines in medicine, even though it has little to nothing in common with them. Let's have a little fireside chat about psychiatry, diagnosing, and the bible of mental illness.

Chapter 2:

Mental Health/Mental Illness, Diagnosing, and Drugs

To understand the field of "mental health" or "mental illness," you must understand the study of psychology and the discipline of psychiatry and all its disciples, e.g., psychotherapists, social workers, psychologists, and the like. Psychiatry mimics other medical disciplines including family medicine, endocrinology, etc. Psychiatry and all its disciples are all based in philosophy, which is simply the art of hypothesizing about human behavior and the world around us. There is no real systematic scientific method and data that backs it up. Unfortunately, those who are not well-versed in, or part of, the system have no idea. Psychology purports to use the scientific method to prove a plethora of hypotheses. However, it only mimics the others using the actual scientific method. I will mention this again, however the best example of how unscientific psychology and psychiatry are is that Freud was rejected 13 times for the Nobel Prize. Why? His work was not scientifically based. Think about this and how all that followed in one way or another was modeled after his work, up to and including the current trauma fad.

My first inkling of this was when I did my first psychological research in graduate school. I wanted to prove or disprove that high school girls' choices of careers had changed. I systematically drew up a "non-biased" survey and then distributed it to all the high schools in the city where I was living. Lo and behold, as I tallied the results—systematically, of course—the results showed there was no change. Then lo and behold, as I tallied the data, I could slant the results whichever way I wanted and still be following the rules for legitimate research. The same was apropos for the "tool" I had developed under the supervision of my esteemed professors. Hopefully, the research for the coronavirus is not using this type of "scientific method." Hopefully, no one will stake their lives on any psychological research.

Psychology remains true to its philosophical roots. We observe the world around us and want it to make sense, just as the philosophers in ancient Greece and Rome would have done. I recall one research project just prior to WWII that looked at human contact and babies. The "researcher" looked at babies in an orphanage and instructed the caretakers not to touch a group of them. Lo and behold, they found the death rate higher for the "untouched" babies. A shocking experiment with the outcome the researchers had expected, of course. The problem is that you can't put babies or any humans in a petri dish and get hard scientific data. The field will not acknowledge this, but it is the truth.

Again, research in psychology is developmentally at the same stage as when philosophers declared the world was flat. It does not have the hard scientific data and method to declare the world is round. One example of this was the scientifically based diagnosis of homosexuality. The same method applies to all manner of diagnosing in psychiatry and its disciples. I did research many years after grad school about parenting and mental health with Boston University. I had the same problem. I could turn the results any way I wished. Lo and behold, outcomes were consistent with the original hypothesis!

The actual science we have about the human brain is very limited. We have progressed a small step beyond when, in the not-too-distant past, psychology lauded phrenology the study of the bumps on your head. A wonderful book, *The Future Mind*, does outline what limited progress has been made. I would suggest you read it before getting involved in any psychiatric treatment. For example, we do know that when the central nervous system is triggered to produce serotonin, we feel great, on top of the world—put more succinctly: "high."

The pharmaceutical industry has used this piece of information to boost sales, and the psychiatric industry has responded well to the impetus by drug companies. Unfortunately, the plethora of antidepressants generally do not have this effect. So, sales are good only because of the "placebo effect" and customers trying one drug after the other looking for a magic pill to fix depression.

This is another piece of the puzzle. In the U.S.A., our mentality is that we want instant gratification, and we want the problem fixed yesterday. What better place to pedal psychiatric drugs? Unfortunately, if you read the side effects, but who has time? The side effects are the same symptoms that you want to get rid of.

An added benefit is that the drug companies supply the staff pushing the drugs with free luncheons, workshops in scenic places, and so on. I thought this had become illegal until I recently went into the lunchroom and found a lovely spread, courtesy of our drug rep. Another testament to the power of money, lobbyists, and our government. Money talks, truth walks—or, at least, is pushed under the proverbial rug. As an aside, it was observed in a psychiatric ward that the antidepressant drug Wellbutrin could cause people to quit smoking. So then it was prescribed for this. Picture the added profits! I have never met a person for whom this has worked. It is a very good example of the "scientific method" in psychiatry. A very good example of the ruthlessness for profit by the drug industry.

Let's say you have decided that one of these antidepressant miracle drugs is just the ticket for you, but after some time, the side effects become more annoying than the problem or create more problems, such as depression, weight gain, suicidal tendencies, etc. So you start titrating off the drug. To refresh your memory, this means to take smaller and smaller doses to wean off something. Now, we have yet another problem. The symptoms that you originally took the drug for and/or the effects of the drug get worse and worse as you titrate down. So what is a psychiatrist or a nurse to do? Increase the dosage, of course! Now you are stuck in the eternal cycle of the use of psychopharmacological drugs. If you have found a drug that cured your symptoms, please stay on it. You are a rare and unique individual.

This is a brief introduction into the world of psychiatric drugs. You need to be properly diagnosed, of course, to be prescribed the appropriate drug that will cure you. Just like when you get strep throat, right? Not so much.

Let's explore the world of psychiatric diagnosing, shall we? To begin, I can assure you that you can go to five different "treaters" and get five different diagnoses, unless they are being lazy and just copy one off your record. The DSM is the holy bible of diagnosing, but I can assure you, it offers no miracles. It has a catchy scientific-sounding title, and I can also assure you that that is where the science ends. The title stands for Diagnostic and Statistical Manual of Mental Health Disorders. When it became hard to ignore the fact that psychiatric diagnoses were helter-skelter and in no way scientifically or statistically based, a very bright and, pardon my saying, a very manipulative psychiatrist came up with the idea of the DSM about 30 years ago. We are now into the fifth edition. Originally, it was to be reviewed every few years. You can see this did not happen.

As an aside, I saw research recently done at Cambridge University. The findings of the research said serotonin has no relationship to depression. The antidepressant drugs generally are based on the concept that lack of serotonin causes depression, so these drugs flood your system with serotonin. Is it no surprise that the folks I have worked with over many years consistently report no effect from these drugs as they were tried on one brand after another and as doses were increased to the maximum level?

The last system of diagnosing used a series of "axes" to delineate the patient's level of mental illness. It gave the opportunity for more than one diagnosis and more than one axis to describe how incapacitated a person was. This was a number that was pretty much arbitrarily picking one that you liked. The new and improved method uses codes instead. I am not privy as to why the change. Perhaps they needed revenue in book sales, since you had to purchase a new DSM to have the codes for varying and important purposes, such as billing insurance companies. The diagnosis continued to be as arbitrary and unscientific as previously. Prior editions were simply amended, including no longer using homosexuality as a mental illness and renaming manic-depressive disorder to bipolar disorder, for example.

It was quite revealing when the push was on to diagnose children as bipolar. Then, the array of drugs previously only for adult use could be used on children. I was quite surprised the other day when a representative of my Department of Mental Health asked for the patient's DSM axis 1 and axis 2 diagnosis. Didn't he get the memo back in 2014, almost seven years ago? Perhaps they can't afford the new version? DMH positions generally are paid more than those of us in private nonprofits, and we must always buy our own copy. I make this point because diagnosing your friends and family can be a fun game, but it is the use of diagnoses, with all the horrendous ramifications that ensue, that wreaks havoc in many, many lives.

As I just mentioned, programs and most services use the DSM labels as gateway devices and ways of controlling spending on needed services. I would think that a person feeling that he or she needs the services would be enough. I had the experience recently of referring a person to a program that I had been instrumental in starting and running. A young man whom I had referred to and knew could benefit greatly from the program was seen to have the "wrong" diagnosis per DMH mandates. Keep in mind what I mentioned previously, in that they were still using the system, as questionable as it is, which was outdated seven years ago. Money talks.

Having started the program, I asked them what diagnosis they would like. As an aside, one of the tenets of the program is that you are not a diagnosis, and they do not matter. So, with the flick of a pen or the computer, miracles of miracles, the young man was given a diagnosis so he could access the services that will help him recover. Will miracles never cease?

The issue is that those working on behalf of the bureaucracy or DMH generally have worked in the field but went on to greener pastures for greener money. Who can blame them? How about we put the money into reputable programs and skip DMH and the mental health centers? I am certain this will not happen in my lifetime, but it has been proven time and time again that the best programs are not under the auspices of mental health centers or DMH.

In conclusion, let me summarize, because I know this information might be new and probably unsettling. Again, if you are happy with the system and have been diagnosed in a way that provides you with drugs you enjoy or that have rid you of your symptoms, perhaps there is no reason for you to read on. Those in the former group are numerous, in the latter group are few to none. You get diagnosed via the DSM, which has no scientific basis. The proof is in the plethora of diagnoses you get that generally increase with the number of providers you see. The pretense of making up the DSM was to resolve this problem. It becomes a catch-22 situation, as there is no scientific basis for the DSM, so there is no consistency. Period. None. No scientific basis at all.

Keep in mind that in any branch of medicine, the reason that anyone is diagnosed is to prescribe treatment and resolve the problem. This NEVER happens in psychiatry and all its minions. So let's see, if you were previously diagnosed as homosexual then supplied with whatever drugs or treatment psychiatry prescribes, then you must be cured. I think this example will help you understand the lack of science and how what is socially cool or uncool at the time will determine what is or is not an illness and what is or is not treatment.

One of the diagnoses made up about 30 years ago was borderline personality disorder. When I first heard it, I thought hmmm … does it mean the person is on the verge of having a personality? This was interesting, as I observed that 99% of the folks diagnosed with this disorder were women. I asked myself, why, in a culture where women's power was generally limited, many would manipulate to get their way. A man using women brags about it. A woman using men is labeled as having borderline personality or worse. More on this later, when we get into the whole area of "diagnosing" a personality disorder. Is it mental health or moral health?

Shall we call antisocial behavior mental illness or moral illness? There is an entire section in the DSM that was fabricated for such situations. The founding attorney for this thinking was brilliant and sleazy. When you need to get someone off, turn despicable behavior into an illness. Brilliant! Unfortunately, the outcome for those who truly suffer has been stigma. No one pays attention to research data that has repeatedly said that mental illness does not make anyone more violent or, shall we say, antisocial. More discussion later separating what are now called personality disorders from all other diagnoses.

A deadlier use of fabricated diagnosis is to prescribe for you the drug or treatment that will "fix" you. At the beginning of my career, I met a man who had one of psychiatry's innovative cures; it was called a lobotomy. I still remember with sadness the scars on his head, the vacant eyes, and the vegetable person this produced. Electroshock therapy is currently done on the unwinnable cases of depression and/or those not responding to the miracle drugs or "15 minutes of fame" they have once a month with a psychiatrist and now, more likely a nurse. I watched a vibrant woman who had graduated from the same university I had be turned into someone whose only way of communicating was to repeatedly ask me, "Am I okay?" No, Jean, you are not okay, and neither is the system that caused this. What was done to you and continues to be done is not okay.

The key to appropriate diagnosing, then, is providing the appropriate treatment, which, when translated, means some type of psychopharmacological intervention which, when translated, means drugs. There are many, and they are constantly reproducing. Who does it benefit? When the karma is correct, and Mars is well-aligned, it benefits the patient, but without fail, it's the drug companies that benefit. It amazes me that there has been a major outcry about the "opioid crisis" and barely a peep about the psychiatric drug tsunami. Many of these drugs are bigger on the street than pain pills ever dreamed of being.

Let's talk about a couple of drugs that are quite popular, both in the office and on the street: Klonopin and Adderall. Many folks coming to your neighborhood mental health center are coming for these types of drugs. The game plan is that to receive these, the patient must come in for one therapy session a month. They see a psychiatrist or, what is more common, the nurse, as nurses are a bit cheaper and easier to come by. The phenomenon within the mental health field, as in other branches of medicine, is that treatment is no longer driven by the professionals. It is driven by the insurance companies. How much "therapy" can be done by one session monthly? None, of course. I assume that the one-session rule is to thwart any legal problems before they arise, since the patient is getting therapy along with their prescription, and any lawyer can attest to it.

Another related phenomenon was the push for "short-term therapy," which was initiated by the insurance companies. For what purpose? For the purpose of the insurance companies having to pay for fewer sessions. This is more of a push with the private companies like Blue Cross. What was equally revealing was the push by graduate schools, with a corresponding course called "Short-Term Therapy."

I have a client who obviously is very fond of Klonopin, and the push now is to reduce doses to avoid addiction. Too little, too late for this woman. She has been on it many years and is clearly addicted. She recently found out that she is in kidney failure. There is a certain mentality that if it's being prescribed by a doctor—or now, the new trend, by a nurse—then it won't be addictive. Other things like heroin and cocaine are, but NOT prescription drugs. Keep in mind that heroin and cocaine were once available by prescription and OTC. Anyway, when the nurse lowered her dose just a bit, she recounted how she was "curled up in a ball in a fetal position, overwhelmed with anxiety and depression." I guess the nurse got tired of arguing and put the dose back up to the prior level. The client was immediately cured. Miracles do happen. As an aside, this person died from kidney failure.

One other example of this "scientific method" of diagnosing and then supplying with the appropriate treatment, i.e., drug, is the use of Adderall. One of the biggest pushers of Adderall is to be found on any college or university campus. What student who has procrastinated studying during the entire semester would not welcome a magic pill that allows them to accomplish in a night or two what should have been done all semester long? The Rolling Stones sang the virtue of "mother's little helper" years ago, so it's nothing new. Freud used cocaine for his unconscious a century ago, so again, nothing new. What is new is that we want immediate easy cures and fail to acknowledge that people are different in terms of abilities. What is new is the massive use of the drug for folks "fortunate" enough to be diagnosed with ADHD and its many counterparts.

To refer you back to the art of diagnosing, being labeled ADHD is as legitimate as being labeled homosexual. Do you have problems focusing? Can't sit still? Perhaps have had less-than-adequate grades? Then ADHD is the label for you, and ADHD drugs will fix this problem immediately. Unfortunately, the high from Adderall is as desirable as any of the "gateway" drugs. The reality is that we can only concentrate five to fifteen minutes at a time. We are not created equally.

If we turn what is average or normal into an illness or disability, the possibilities are endless. And the possibilities of prescription drugs as gateway drugs are also endless. If you have a predilection for upping the dosage due to desire or addiction, this leaves many in the position of doctor shopping or buying on the street to increase their dosage.

The reality also is that we are all victims of the bell curve. There is a very small percentage who have laser and lengthy ability to focus and the discipline not to procrastinate important tasks. We all fall somewhere on the continuum, and the rush to develop a pill to address or fix your "problem," which is normal, has resulted in a tsunami of drugs and billions of dollars to the pharmaceutical industry. Unfortunately, many parents, teachers, and mental health professionals are more than happy to purchase this myth. The price to be paid for this is currently being calculated, as was the price of opioids previously.

To conclude our study of diagnosing and prescribing, I will offer you a real-life example that touches upon all the points I have made. The example is of a young person, who wishes to remain anonymous, and I assure you that it is a very real example, as are the endless examples brewing as I write this. The young person in question had been a stellar student in grammar school, high school, and college. He was an honor student, member of the National Honor Society, captain of several sports teams, leader of the drama club and member of jazz and other music clubs, to name a few of his accomplishments. Please make note, as having academic difficulties is the hallmark of an ADHD diagnosis. So there is no confusion, to be awarded the ADHD diagnosis, there would be a history of academic issues and an inability to do well in school.

This young person proceeded on to college and perhaps became more interested in partying and sports activities than in studying. So all one needs to do is to go to your local college clinic and secure a supply of Adderall, which he did, with the full support of a family member with a history of addiction that included illegal substances comparable to Adderall. The young person with endless potential had been pushed into the addiction rabbit hole by family and psychiatry. It was the beginning of the end and came within a hair's breadth of ending him. He ascended to the heights in a profession that is incredibly competitive. He descended just as quickly, leaving the family praying moment to moment that the dreaded call in the middle of the night would not come.

Finally, he returned home so swollen by drugs that he could barely fit in the back seat of the car. When he was refused what he demanded, his response was to nail the doors shut so no one could leave the house. Finally, with a bit of tough love by those who love but were not so tough, he began the journey called recovery.

The first major death-affirming tactic was brought into play by his then-psychiatrist. The psychiatrist was fully apprised of his Adderall addiction. The fully apprised psychiatrist then prescribed, guess what! Adderall. The plunge towards certain death began again. The whole attempted murder landed in drug court, which could have provided an answer. The DSM-thumping, Adderall-pushing psychiatrist testified that the young man was not addicted but mentally ill, so no drug court for him. More like no lawsuit for Mr. Psychiatrist, as why would a competent doctor supply an addict with the drug of his choice? Mr. Psychiatrist had found his loophole, his defense. They settled later out of court. The damage was done.

The most recent scam by the pharmaceutical companies is prescribing Gabapentin as being non-addictive. It is highly addictive.

Chapter 3:

Beyond the Myth of Mental Health – It's Mental Health, Not Moral Health

A cautionary word, particularly to those beginning their journey as a therapist, social worker, psychiatric nurse, etc. You don't fix anyone; they fix themselves. You can be a caring, supportive partner with them, but in the end, recovery is not something done to anyone. It is something done with them. The other "culturally relevant" concept is that human beings are diverse and have a wide range of behaviors. This does not make them ill; it just makes them different. We are quick to diagnose, as diagnosing will give us the cure. Not so much in psychiatry. It may open the floodgates for teachers, parents, and psychiatrists to foist medication on unsuspecting children. It will open the floodgates for psychiatrists, nurses, and therapists to open the floodgates on unsuspecting adults. Why? Not for the benefit of the child, but a drugged child is certainly less troublesome for the adults in charge. The adult will also be stupefied, making them a lot less troublesome to others involved in their lives. If they fail to cooperate, there is always the mandatory order called a "Rogers." Just so you are aware, this is a legal order that can force anyone to take psychiatric medication against their will.

All adults are different. All children are different. Shall we embrace these differences? No, we shall diagnose them, since embracing them is a lot more work. For the child, generally male, his problem sitting still and focusing is a major challenge for the adults around him. How about we change the system, as opposed to changing him? How about we do things like reinstituting multiple recesses to calm him down? How about we give him tutors to help him focus? How about we at least recognize and try to address what is usually a chaotic home life filled with serial fathers or mothers, drugs, abuse, marriages that are conflicted, or whatever else, as opposed to diagnosing him as ADHD? We can't force these families to change—just ask any DCF worker—but we can be more effective with our methods to engage, set limits, and educate.

This concept of the "range of behaviors" goes back to Freud and his cohorts. Yes, it is illness for the child with very limited verbal and cognitive abilities. No, it is not illness for the child often living in dysfunction in school and at home. The child is coping very well but not in the eyes of most of the adults around him or her. The home, school, and mental health system all collude so the answer suits the system and the adults, not the child. All children are not created equal. Some are verbal, and some are not. Some can sit for periods of time, and some cannot.

But to address whatever situation is causing the problems will take time, creativity, and, more importantly in our culture, money. So we go for the cheap, easier, uncreative shortcut because it's easier on everyone except the child. We "diagnose" them with contrived diagnoses that fit perfectly with this "model of treatment." The naturally athletic child will run with ease. The child who is not will need much coaching and will never perform with the same ease as the child with this innate ability. The old heredity vs. environment debate is not dead.

We have become a culture where what are normal behaviors are now illnesses. What are differences are now illnesses, with all the accompanying stigma and drugs to use.

Another concept is that of "personality disorders." This and the "not guilty by reason of insanity" legal modus operandi have been the biggest promoters of stigma. To classify a group of folks struggling with anxiety, depression, delusions, or hallucinations as immoral law breakers due to these symptoms, just because at some point an attorney said it was so, is gravely immoral. People who break the law are just that: people who break the law. There is no correlation between this and mental illness. It is a last-ditch effort by lawyers who have run out of tricks. And yes, there are people who struggle with mental illness who break the law and some who are immoral, but no greater number than those who don't have a diagnosis and break the law. If we treat all with dignity and compassion when we arrest them, perhaps we can alleviate many problems. Innocent until proven guilty. A person diagnosed wielding a weapon is no more lethal than one not diagnosed.

As I had mentioned, the diagnosis of "borderline personality disorder" is one of the more recently contrived contributions to the personality disorders. Could we perhaps see these women—and it is almost always women—as trying to make it in the world? When you don't have power, manipulation is the next best thing. Perhaps as sexism in our culture decreases, the borderline label will be deleted, as has been done with many others. The system is not scientific but it is stigmatizing and sexist. Perhaps as the diagnosis of homosexual was recently deleted, we can do the same with borderline. And maybe we can also delete transvestite.

So what are the symptoms we need to treat? Anxiety, depression, hallucinations, and delusions. The area of addiction is another issue. The field of mental health has been the biggest promoter of addiction. Some can take the psychiatric drugs and get an ongoing and pleasant high. Others with a predisposition for addiction will be sent into a black hole again. The opioid crisis is a minor storm in comparison to the tsunami approaching via psychiatric drugs. The mental health field needs to extricate itself from the role of promoting dependence and addiction.

Let's start with anxiety. If you think about it, addressing a person's anxiety is about helping them get through it with their active involvement. Often, we are promoting the symptom and the illness. I often meet people who are afraid to leave their house; call it agoraphobia if you will. Perhaps the person has no reason, desire, or motivation to leave their house. They are getting all they need at home, and the world can be an awful, scary place. One person said she missed going to her daughter's events; however, it was not a strong enough motivator for her to want to change this behavior. It is my judgment that it is important for her to go to these events, not hers. Who's crazy now?

Dealing with anxiety and recovery is hard work. You can't will it to be so. I recently heard rumors that a new and very cool diagnosis is in the works. Some children and adults eat a very limited variety of foods. Always a battle, to be sure, but to expedite things, we can create an illness around this particular anxiety and behavior, as has been done with a plethora of other behaviors, such as shyness becoming autism. This also grants absolution from responsibility to the caregiver. Most of the kids I see diagnosed with autism, ADHD, and other comparable labels represent dysfunctional families, character traits that should be accepted and not turned into so-called illnesses. I said most, as there are children who are truly autistic, and we all recognize them when we meet them. And most families are dysfunctional.

I guarantee you that whatever anxiety you have and wish not to allow to ruin your life can be resolved. If we establish a trusting relationship, if you want to progress, you will recover. Of course, there are drugs for this, but proceed at your own risk. If you have the propensity for addiction, they can send you down a black hole rather quickly. If the drug is labeled one of the "bad" drugs, you will be taken off abruptly. This, in combination with a propensity for addiction, spells disaster. When you try to get off these drugs, your anxiety increases.

If it is not labeled as one of the bad drugs, your nurse or doctor will then increase the dosage. Now you are a gerbil on the wheel and a product of the mental health system promoting patienthood. If you look at the plethora of diagnoses in the DSM, anxiety is always a symptom. We can treat anxiety without using contrived diagnoses, prescribing meds that are a hit-or-miss proposition, promoting stigma, and making people dependent on the "system."

The next symptom that can also be successfully treated is depression. This is described as problems with sleeping, fatigue, appetite, sadness, and suicidal thoughts. As an aside, I googled depression to make certain I did not miss any of the symptoms. You never know; this changes with the wind. And what to my wandering eyes should appear? "Trintellix." Just the drug to cure your depression or "increase your suicidal thoughts," whichever comes first, I guess.

The thing I have always found scariest is suicide. It frightened me to death when I first began this work many centuries ago and still does. I am responsible for this person's well-being and safety. As I have mentioned, you don't do "helping" to someone. They need to choose to be helped. After that choice is made, the helper needs to jump in with both feet to help in any way possible. This brings up what I always have thought was a very dysfunctional perspective. Many of my fellow therapists and managers of said therapists are clear that there is therapy, and there is case management, and never the twain shall meet.

Case management is generally viewed as the lowlier of the two jobs, since it can be done by folks with no degree or "just a BA" degree. The loftier job of psychotherapy needs at least a master's degree AND, added on later, the appropriate license. The license thing is recent and just as scientific as the DSM, which means it is not scientific at all. When I began this work, there were no licenses. The reality is that a license and whatever the arbitrary criteria are have nothing to do with a therapist doing a good job.

So how do you prevent someone from killing themselves? The honest answer is that you don't. This by no means insinuates that you do not do everything humanly possible to prevent it, but ultimately, this is the individual's choice. It is well-known that people who suicide "successfully" often never said a word. The term "successful suicide" shows you probably better than anything else how very dysfunctional psychiatry and its disciples are. How can anyone label a person who is desperate enough to kill themselves as "successful"? Having had a near-death experience, it is my job to help the person want to stay here and not leave out of desperation.

So, how do you do this? You care genuinely with no power plays stated or insinuated. How do most of us figure out if someone cares? By their sitting there for 50 minutes and nodding empathetically at us? No, usually the lowly art of case management somehow comes into play. Do you think a person, or client, or patient thinks that you care if you ignore the fact that they are homeless and/or may not have enough to eat? My guess is probably not.

Common sense tells us that we should stay tuned in to the hints that people may drop if they are thinking about killing themselves. However, this is not an intervention per se or way to stop them from "successfully" killing themselves. You must genuinely care and genuinely help meet their needs. So many times, I have had folks tell me after the fact that it was all planned, means secured, and they had no intention of saying anything but realized that some caring action had stopped them at least in that moment. You can't "fake it until you make it." You must truly care, and this is not a teachable skill. You either do or don't. If you don't, find another profession. As you can see, this can truly be a matter of life and death. Something that contributes is the constant barrage of the media where everyone is happy, beautiful, and fulfilled.

Chapter 4:

Can You Cure Mental Illness?

Yes! There you have it. Yes, you can cure mental illness. It sounds simple and straightforward, but it is not. Addiction you cannot cure, but you can put it into remission. There are three categories: addiction, mental health challenges, and personality disorders. This does not mean that anyone in any of these groups can't suffer from symptoms labeled as mental health challenges.

It is time that we stop stigmatizing and giving a life sentence to those who struggle with anxiety, depression, and psychosis. There are times when folks recover and are cured. Does that mean they will never again have a problem? No. Some do, and some don't. If you recover from strep throat and are cured, does that mean you will never get strep throat again? The perspective that people cannot be cured is a boon to the pharmaceutical industry, but beyond that, it has no real purpose except stigmatizing those who have suffered. If you have broken your leg and then it has healed, are you required to use crutches for the rest of your life for fear of falling? Why do we do this with problems of the mind, where our knowledge and understanding are the least? Perhaps that is part of the reason. It is because we do not have the knowledge to truly understand and treat, so we relegate the patient to the status of eternal patient.

The dynamics of the use of psychotropic meds is yet another testament to the need by the psychiatric community to keep folks as eternal patients and never cured. I owe some of my understanding of this to Chaya Grossberg. Thank you, Chaya. She said, and I have also found this to be true, that when you attempt to go off most psychiatric meds, the symptoms get worse.

Another piece of information is: Read the side effects. Generally, they are the same symptoms you are trying to get rid of. Again, our lack of understanding and knowledge leaves us with little to no understanding. It used to be that when a person was being taken off medication or having a change in medication, they would be hospitalized. In our world, where the insurance companies and not the doctors are making medical decisions, this process is expected to happen in the doctor's office. Chaya, on her website, speaks of how devastating this process is. So, as the doctor and patient are working this out and the symptoms get worse, what is the response? The response of most if not all psychiatric providers is to then increase the dosage.

We all have anxiety. If life is going as we want it to, then anxiety is our friend and made to protect us from harm. When life events get out of control, so can anxiety. Does this mean it will last forever? No, but in our culture, we want immediate relief, so we take a pill. Many of the triggers for anxiety are outside of the home. Some folks begin decreasing their time outside of the home for this reason, and then many of the activities that give their life meaning disappear. And so depression and isolation set in.

The people I have met who have been labeled agoraphobic are those who have ended up being captives in their own home. When you first choose not to leave, the process snowballs, and it becomes harder and harder to leave. But I also hear from some agoraphobic patients who will casually mention that they went to the store since they needed food or attended a child's baptism because they couldn't miss that, etc. Like medication, once into this loop, it becomes more and more difficult to leave. But as you see, if someone is motivated, it's still possible.

So, what is the option? If they get the proper help and/or motivate themselves, they can return to a normal level of anxiety, which means they still have it, of course, and there will still be events that trigger major increases. The difference is that they have taught themselves or have had someone else teach them how to cope. They are, in fact, cured.

The problem is that when they seek help from their local mental health center, they can get pushed into a lifetime of illness as opposed to a cure. If you demand that this problem go away immediately, take a pill. If you think there won't be times when anxiety is high, stay in your house. If you think you can continue to function, congratulations. You have cured yourself.

I have experienced this professionally and personally. I guarantee you that choosing to work through it is your best option. Again, anxiety will always be there. It will ebb, and it will flow. As you learn ways to deal with it, you are, in fact, cured. Keep in mind, we are all unique. Being cured of strep throat does not mean you will never catch it again. It is our attitude and the system that give us the idea that mental health problems are never cured. Keep in mind, all the diagnoses in the DSM are fabricated. Made up with no scientific basis.

So what purpose do the DSM and diagnosing serve? As patients, we are taught that if you have the correct diagnosis, then you will be cured. In other medical disciplines, this usually is the case—with exceptions, of course. The psychiatric patient feels better if they are labeled and then either denies or gets confused when they are given 10 different diagnoses by 10 different diagnosers. There will be more consistency if the diagnosers read the record, of course. The psychiatrist and more often now, the nurse, will then throw a drug cocktail at them hoping something will "stick." Keep in mind that psychiatry grew out of philosophy. If you remember that, it is easier to see how psychiatric diagnosing is conjecture and not science.

What about depression? Can it be cured? Yes. If you doubt that psychiatric treatment is dubious, just watch the field for a few years. The latest "new and improved" approach is always there. When I started out, we had reality therapy, behavioral therapy, and psychoanalytic therapy. Today, the vogue is everything cognitive and traumatic. DBT, CBT, trauma this and trauma that. Wasn't it Freud who said that the first major trauma is separation anxiety, which causes a lifetime of psychosis and/or neurosis? No cure there, for sure. Shall we continue to promote this? Or perhaps it is time for some honesty and a change.

I just saw on 60 Minutes that the "new and cutting-edge therapy" is a psychiatrist using psychedelic drugs on his patients. We have been this way before. Remember Timothy Leary and the resulting cases of disaster? Freud was a genius in his time, but perhaps it is time to move ahead. I will outline the things that do work. Generally, the latest dog-and-pony show will borrow a piece of what we all know does work and combine it with some intricate and bizarre method that they contend never fails.

Depression, like anxiety, is part of who we are. In the psychiatric world, depression and anxiety walk hand in hand. If you look at what we call the "symptoms" of depression, generally, it describes any one of us at any point in time. Disruptions in sleep? Eating? Relationships? Feelings of sadness? Isolation? Lack of interest? The problem becomes a problem when you decide that it IS a problem. Like anxiety, we all function (or not) daily with some combination of these "symptoms." Another issue in psychiatry is that psychiatry has turned everything into an illness. As I had mentioned, I chuckled recently as I read a proposal by a psychologist that it is imperative that the fact that some folks have limited food choices be turned into a diagnosis. What next? How about those with limited choices of what color they wear? Black is my only choice, and you know what THAT means.

Depression has become a major focus for the pharmaceutical industry, and given that we all have it, this will bring them megabucks. So to accommodate this "need," they have produced thousands of these ineffective antidepressant drugs to increase the profit margin. I have yet to meet anyone who has told me that they have taken an antidepressant and been cured; it usually reflects the same impact a placebo would give. Generally, they report that they have tried three or four or nine or 10 different drugs, and usually they don't work. This is not surprising, given our current level of understanding of the brain and central nervous system. Read the fine print. Most if not all these ads say the scientific information is little to none. Some say they have found one that works, which is perhaps the placebo effect or a random roll of the biological dice. Getting up out of bed and going to work, the gym, or whatever can be easier if you have a cheering section. Notice how unscientific the indices for depression are.

Sleep disruption—if normally you get up once during the night, and this becomes twice, does this make you ill? If you lost your puppy a month ago and are still feeling sad, does this make you ill? If you are in bed all day and can't get up, chances are, you won't find a therapist to make house calls. So by the time you have gotten out of bed, made an appointment, gotten dressed, and made it to the appointment, you are well on your way to recovery. If you are functioning and have bouts of sadness, overeating, and sleeplessness, join the crowd. You only become officially ill when you make it to the therapist and are diagnosed, as you MUST be diagnosed for the insurance company to pay. Keep in mind where and how diagnoses are fabricated. How ironic, since it looks like by then, you are halfway to being "cured." However, when you get there, you will generally be told what sad shape you are in. Being depressed, you will readily agree. Can your depression become an illness? Yes. Can depression be cured? Yes. Who decides when you are cured or, shall we say, in balance for you? Is life a straight road? No.

The next symptom that will lead you to be diagnosed, this time in a BIG way, is hallucinations. Hallucinations can affect any of your senses: taste, touch, smell, sight, and hearing. Chances are, you have hallucinated. Have you ever felt someone touch you, turned around, and there was no one there? You probably were having a tactile hallucination. Did you ever taste something and it tasted awful, when others thought it tasted great? You were hallucinating. Did you ever walk into a room and "smell something" when no one else does? This is called an olfactory hallucination. Did you ever see something out of the corner of your eye only to turn and see nothing there? Did you ever hear faint whispers or water running only to discover that no one or nothing is there? Perhaps this auditory hallucination happened for a time or just once and has not happened again. You have been cured of your hallucinations.

Funny how things are culturally defined in that some cultures see hallucinating as a blessing and a sign that you are a deity. In the good ole USA. admitting to hallucinations will get you labeled a "major wacko." The drugs for neurosis are called minor tranquilizers, and those for psychosis are called major tranquilizers. Neurosis will bring you minor stigma, and psychosis will bring you major stigma. So is it not surprising that people go into a major panic when they first experience hallucinations? Can hallucinations be cured? Yes. Can they return? Yes. Is there a pill that will cure hallucinations? No. Do hallucinations tend to disappear with age? Yes.

I had the privilege of meeting and attending a workshop presented by Pat Deigan. Pat, like many folks, earned her doctorate and was on faculty at BU. If I recall correctly, Pat had ended up at one of the state hospitals and eventually gained notoriety for her insightful workshops. This was a time when there was a great push to understand the impact of physical disability. There was a workshop where all able-bodied folks were put into a wheelchair and told to negotiate. This was before curb cuts, ramps, etc.

Pat used a tape recorder with ear phones to simulate hearing voices. She then told workshop participants to go about their normal daily activities. For example, someone might attempt to pick up meds at cvs with "voices" blaring in their ears. The potential using virtual reality and Pat's method would be endless. You could virtually perhaps put someone in a classroom with the voices playing. This would help others develop a true understanding of what "hearing voices" actually feels like. In addition, the use of virtual reality could also help engage adolescents and children who are difficult to engage in standard "talk therapy". Current methods of art therapy and play therapy are helpful. With some imagination and creativity virtual reality could take this to a new level.

Do folks who have hallucinated ever get cured? The answer is yes. Most have a drug cocktail that may or may not help. The initial trauma of hallucinating results in an understandable phobia of changing anything. Initially, people who are hallucinating are uncertain about what are the voices and what is reality. The voices can say some ugly things. I have yet to meet anyone who has had hallucinations explained to them and said that hallucinations caused them to do harm.

This often becomes the perfect legal defense, with the person being coached that this is the way to solve their legal problems. That it's the voices that told them to do it with the implication that they had no control. The psychological research that has remained steady is that "crazy people" are no more violent than "normal people." Of course, there are folks in BOTH groups who are violent. The why of this is another psychiatric unknown. Often, the lack of knowledge in psychiatry results in blaming the patient or, better yet, the patient's mother.

How about delusions? Just because we do not know what will get rid of them does not mean a person cannot be cured of delusions. What I have seen with delusions is that the person can learn not to share this information, and when they do go away, learn also not to share this information due to embarrassment and stigma. A wise choice. Do all people get cured of delusions? Some do, and some don't.

These are what I would label as true psychiatric symptoms. When we get into the area of personality disorders, this is a different story. Can people be cured of personality disorders? Yes. It is a different process to change who you are as opposed to dealing with a symptom. I am certain that the personality disorder, or borderline personality disorder, came about by a disgusted psychiatrist who was probably outwitted by a female patient. As an aside, it is interesting that currently, I see post after post about narcissism. This tells us much about our culture as opposed to telling us about an individual.

Let me discuss the diagnosis of borderline personality. This diagnosis was made up about 30 years ago. I think, since it was fabricated that long ago, I have run into only one male who was diagnosed as borderline. Who knows, with the shift towards gender equality, the number will probably increase. The gist of this diagnosis is women getting or trying to get what they want. Being manipulative works well when you are in an unequal power relationship. Giving someone this diagnosis is the same as the proverbial slap in the face. Knuckle under, ladies—and perhaps gentlemen. If you don't, this diagnosis will be your reprimand to announce to the world how awful you are. So there! Can these ladies be cured? Of course. If they want to change themselves and learn other methods for making their way. As you can see, this is not the same as curing anxiety, etc.

Addiction, which is rampant in our country, must produce certain behaviors for the person to survive. Addiction happens because there is some biochemical reaction that is set off, and initially, the person and any professionals are unaware of this. Nicotine is the deadliest and the most orchestrated. Anyone who is predisposed and tries this drug is addicted almost immediately. I have frequently had heroin addicts tell me that they can quit heroin, but they can't quit smoking. The tobacco companies know what they are doing. Too bad the drug companies aren't as adept with their nicotine patches.

With other drugs, it is usually a longer process. We all go into adolescence and young adulthood experimenting, and some come out as addicts. By virtue of how we look at addiction, we produce behavior disorders. The most effective programs for addressing both the biochemical addiction and the personality changes it brings are AA, NA, and the like. There is always the step to make amends to those you have harmed. The disease of denial. Who would want to admit they have manipulated, stolen, and lied to family and friends to achieve their high? Drug-induced personality disorder can be cured as well as the personality disorder that is not drug-induced. Why do some people become addicts, and some don't? This is unknown. Can addicts be cured? Yes, with the stipulation that they do not use substances legal and illegal. Here is where it really gets muddled.

The psychiatric system currently offers—and has for quite a

while—legal drugs to substitute for your illegal drug addiction. It just substitutes one for the other, with no real change except the threat of getting arrested. Not all, but many are on this legal substitute for eternity. I had one woman recently brag about her 30 years of sobriety, adding that she smokes marijuana daily and takes Suboxone along with Klonopin. The psychiatric system will pronounce her cured. Do you see a problem here? I do, and I also see better solutions.

Chapter 5:

Parenting and Mental Illness/ The Cure for Mental Illness

"The toughest job you'll ever love." Long ago, this was the recruitment slogan for the Marines. Thinking about it, this is the perfect slogan for parenting, in a positive way. Not that it always ends up positive, as many times it is the toughest job you will resent, be overwhelmed by, and/or be angry about for any number of reasons. For example, if the other partner is among the missing, or you just plain feel unprepared for the job.

I will let you in on a secret. No one is ever prepared for this. That being the case, there is also a lack of multi-generational and extended family support for parenting in our culture. If you have this, count yourself as blessed. If you have this and the support is not riddled with addiction and mental health malfunction, you have won the lottery. Congratulations, you are one of the lucky few.

As I was saving posts from Facebook, it became apparent that even the parenting basics are no longer basic. As I thought about the families I have worked with, it became clearer that this is the case, and the values in our culture don't support parenting. Look at the mental health system and the drug-pushing—as opposed to parent-supporting and accountability—that has replaced parenting. This fits the financial needs of the drug companies that push for what once were adult-only diagnoses that are now perfect for kids.

The agenda of having the right to "me time" also fits well with drugging kids and giving a parent sabbatical leave. When kids were left to their own devices at home during the pandemic, is it any wonder that academics went down the tubes, and now the mental health crisis is exploding? No, it's not surprising to those of us who have taught and/or done therapy with these kids. The parental job has been relegated to the schools and school staff. Now this is expected, as opposed to what once was a team effort. I will later tell you the story of Alex H. to illustrate my point. Why are school shootings increasing when there's no one at home to monitor the automatic weapons?

I had a woman I am currently working with tell me how frustrated she is with a relative whose child is totally out of control. They sent her to some type of parenting group where she learned the art of negotiating with her child. Unfortunately, all she learned was negotiating, and they forgot about limit-selling.

If she had gone to Facebook, she would have found numerous examples on limit-selling from all different cultural perspectives. We have the Afro-American dad who made his four-year-old leave Walmart abruptly due to a tantrum or, shall we call it, emotional dysregulation? The scene has dad and daughter sitting in the parking lot, "processing" the event. And shall we say he told her that no daughter of his was going to act that way, and she would not go back in the store until she "cleaned up that mess." As he said, "no whoopin' needed." Nice job, Dad.

Along the same lines, we have "The Mommy Answer Lady." That is your average white middle-class mom telling you "how to stop screen addiction." Why do we turn a lack of parenting into addiction? Anyway, her solution is the same as the dad at Walmart has suggested. She is telling all those parents whose kids have run amuck with technology to "take charge" and "be consistent" and "build your relationship" and to have the kids do daily exercises. As an aside, there was a study by Harvard recently that shows how all the ADHD kids were cured by being allowed to run 45 minutes before school and after school. No surprise there either. What is surprising is that many schools have reduced or eliminated recess time to focus on academics. News flash, guys: Kids can't focus on academics unless they are allowed to be physically active.

Hopefully, the Harvard study will remind you of this. The Rebels Project also posts on Facebook about the perfect storm in our culture that brought us to this ugly, soul-wrenching, beyond devastating place. There are no words. The Columbine survivors in their unfathomable horror found what the "secret pill" is for anyone who is devastated. They reached out to each other. As one survivor stated, "The human connection is what saved me."

Seeing a therapist once a week with a referral to the doctor for drugs with all its nuances does not give a message of genuine caring. Therapists with huge caseloads are not about caring. It's about M-O-N-E-Y. An ad on Facebook tells you how you, too, can make seven figures as a therapist! Is your therapist on call like they should be, or is the motivation just the money? Do you think they have a stopwatch and generally abruptly end your session at the 45-minute mark? I had a client recently say her prior therapist told her it was the law to end a session at 50 minutes.

I'll tell you a story of a friend who was always ripe for becoming a professional patient. The way she was describing the services that her long-term therapist was giving her was ridiculous. I kept telling her to find someone new. Her parents, who were lovely people, did not instill self-sufficiency. Fortunately, she found a husband who took on the job for a time, but he passed away, so she turned to the therapist.

One day, I got a surprising call from my friend. She was in the emergency room. I asked her why, presuming she had gotten hit by a car or Gawd knows what. She said she was in a session with her therapist, and the therapist called the cops and had—shall we call her Priscilla?—escorted to the emergency room. Now, if Priscilla were truly in a crisis, a concerned and caring therapist would have escorted Priscilla to the ER herself. However, this would have meant lost revenue for Ms. Therapist since time is money, ergo, she found the perfect solution for her. This approach was obvious when Priscilla recounted to me what was going on in her session. This worked for both of them. The therapist was happy collecting her hourly fee, and Priscilla was happy with her style.

It worked for both Priscilla and her therapist. Beware if your sessions are 45 minutes or an hour long and your therapist ushers you out accordingly. There is no allowance for a difficult or not-so-difficult time. If the therapist doesn't warn you that they might run late at times with another client, watch out. The same courtesy and caring will be extended to you when you are upset, and the alternative is that you, too, will end up being escorted to the ER. If they do not give you ready access to them between sessions, watch out. If Ms. Therapist genuinely cares, she will give you her personal number. I have been doing this for years, and rarely has it been abused.

I digress. Recently, there has been a challenge on TikTok to hit a teacher. It must be "National Hit a Teacher Week." The teachers, of course, are shocked and outraged—rightfully so. Let us look at how this happened. The phenomenon is popular among middle schoolers and some high schoolers, some of whom are 18. These kids could get arrested and end up in big-person court. Who knows?

If the middle schoolers are being watched by parents as they use social media, how could this happen? The answer, of course, is that they are not being watched. Unfortunately, the parental job description has been extended to controlling social media. At the beginning of this era, a friend and I were trying to figure out what to do. It came down to when our kids were allowed to be on social media, one of us would literally be standing behind them. Yes, it certainly did distract from "me time." And no, you can't send them to their room with unlimited access to social media. Again, parenting 101.

Cruising the pages of Facebook, I saw that the hip therapists are using virtual reality. This makes sense because in the past, board games and art have been used. It's just that now kids are preferring to play in virtual reality. Who can blame them? My boss went into a frenzy when I mentioned wanting to use it. Why? I guess she feared I would not do my parental thing (i.e., set limits and choose the game). I tried to assure her that Connect 4, as I understand it, is just reconstructed tic-tac-toe, and I didn't think it would turn the kid into Ted Bundy. It would just be in a controlled limit-setting kind of a way to help to build a relationship with the kids.

Somewhere on Facebook, it said that virtual reality treats patients more effectively, so the insurance companies would pay for it, and it gets rid of anxiety FAST. The insurance companies will love this. Faster means fewer sessions, which means insurance companies spend less. I have found that insurance companies are great at taking your money but not so great at giving it back. As a culture, faster is better. Unfortunately, many of the things that are creative and not harmful are slow. But no time for this, just give us drugs.

Then, as I perused the pages of social media, I saw ACES being treated as the current cure for whatever ails my child. Adverse Childhood Experiences. Who has not had these? Freud built his theory on this, saying that we spend a lifetime trying to overcome having been separated from our moms!

Nothing new here. This is one of the current "dog-and-pony" shows. Ten years from now it will be relegated to the archives or junk pile of psychological theories.

Have you ever heard of "reality therapy," for example? Who doesn't need a dose of reality now and then? The red flag here is that living in and rehearsing these experiences will relegate you to professional patienthood. Life is trauma and that is inescapable. Some have more, and some have less. Some trauma is VERY traumatizing, of course. The choice can be to make peace with it and move on with life. The choice can be to live in it and stay put. The reality is that at a vulnerable time in your life, you can run into therapists who will encourage one or the other. Buyer beware!

A discussion of parenting would not be complete without talking about the most popular diagnoses with the kids today, those being ADHD and on the autism spectrum. Every child has difficulty focusing, particularly boys. Our own ability to focus as adults is generally less than a couple of minutes, and unfortunately, it gets progressively worse. As I mentioned earlier, a Harvard study cured all the ADHD children by letting them run wild twice a day. You take the fact that running wild is the nature of any child, and then you place them in shackles for six hours daily in classrooms that have too many students. Teachers have no help, and parents are not present. What do you get when you put these together? ADHD, of course!

This is a great opportunity to tell you the story of—let's call him Charles. Charles began kindergarten with my daughter at a local private parochial school. She landed there because my son had been lost on his first day of kindergarten when he attended the local public school. Allow me to add that I was and remain a single parent with major medical issues, so you won't think this is a family with time and money to spare. The scenario that will cure ADHD, autism, and Asperger's is parents being willing to do whatever it takes; and teachers truly invested in their work. Since parochial school wages are always low; and classes not being so large that they are unmanageable and where having the most up-to-date equipment is not necessary. In place of this, the public school offers a weekly therapy session and the medication of your choice. This refers to most kids. There are some kids with true limitations.

Charles began kindergarten in a rather notorious way. He was the designated biter in the class, and he ended up biting my daughter. If this had been in your average school, it probably could have resulted in a lawsuit, with Charles being banned at least for a while as he was psychologically "assessed" and prescribed whatever would be conducive for his return.

This is not what happened. Everyone came to assist, including mom and the school. I had met his mom because parents at the school are involved. She was gracious and apologized profusely. Then she went into the classroom regularly to prevent a repeat performance. We all wanted Charles to do well, and eventually, he did. There were many other issues along the way, of course. I saw recently he had completed a master's degree at a prestigious university and was on his way to a professional job and fulfilling life. It was, my guess, that the outcome would have been very different if he had not had the support he did.

I just saw a news program about an innovative program at a school in Shreveport, Louisiana. The program was called "Dads on Duty." (How many dads and moms are off-duty?) A very simple but very powerful premise. There had been ongoing riots at the school. Obviously, the dads got tired of having their kids beaten up and in danger daily, so they started a "Pa Patrol." Every day, a group of dads were present at the school, caring and setting limits. Another way of saying it: parenting the kids who were missing this in their lives—certainly a better parenting device than sending in the police. And guess what!

With the dads present, the riots disappeared, and everyone lived happily ever after. Well, at least there was peace for now, and I am certain that the kids of these dads are doing well. Does anything sound familiar here? I think Dads on Duty and Charles's mom would have a great deal in common if they met.

How about autism? Yes, there are children who are socially limited and need much support. They are not very verbal and often have medical complications like seizures and diabetes as well. They often need extra support and medication. The problem comes in when the idea of a spectrum is presented and there is no line of demarcation. This was previously intertwined with intelligence, and now some children are also diagnosed with ID. However, the child who was once called "shy" is now autistic. What is a personality trait has become a mental illness. We must ask why.

All kids are not created equal or the same. All kids are not socially adept. Just like all children will not be future Olympic champions. Some kids may do well in school, but ask them to build a house or fix a car, and they are lost. What are cultural and individual differences, we have made into an illness. Why? Responsibility. Once you diagnose a child and remember how those are made up, it absolves the adults of responsibility and opens the floodgates for medication. There have always been children who have had to go to the nurse for meds. Do you wonder why the line outside the nurse's office has begun to snake around the building and out the door? I mean this literally.

So what's the answer? To be honest, I don't even know if an answer is possible anymore in the public sector here in the good ol' U.S. of A. As you can see with Charles, some of it was the school, some of it was his family, and the last piece was the other parents in the school. No, it is not all about money. Remember, the teachers in parochial school are paid less.

However, it is about money in that the class sizes are generally smaller. It is about dedication that has no price tag. It is about parenting regardless of the sacrifice and lack of "me time." Most moms are now juggling what is a full-time job and full-time parenting. We have substituted full-time parenting with a prescription pad and 45 minutes a week with an adult. The result has been school shootings, a drug epidemic, and the need for Dads on Duty.

The Final Chapter

We are a culture of quick fixes. Your value is determined by how much wealth you have. Politics are controlled by money. A family can be shattered in a moment by a "quick" divorce. Extended family is available to the select few. People new to this country may have it but will eventually assimilate into the broader culture. Differences are not valued. These differences can be cultural, or having hallucinations, or having ideas different from the mainstream. These outliers will be devalued, ridiculed, jailed, and institutionalized. Kindness and compassion are not what we truly value, and to serve our own benefit, we often target folks demonstrating these qualities. This is the "me world" looking for me time, not we time. If something is "scientifically proven," however, this "research," valid or not, is right, and it is good. Here we have the perfect tsunami for what is labeled mental health "treatment."

It is no surprise that we have school shooters and that drug use is epidemic. The politicians cry that we need more mental health services. Yes, of course we do. What we need the most is to be honest about our reality and a major change in our culture.

The "drug culture" in psychiatry echoes the overall culture and fits in quite nicely. This dynamic is much to the benefit of the pharmaceutical companies with their impressive army of lobbyists. Feeling anxious, depressed, out of sorts? Do I have the drug for you! It is never mentioned that these emotions are part of who we are as humans. You will never be rid of them and experience only euphoric emotions, and this is where the psychiatric drugs come in. The most popular drugs, Klonopin, Adderall, and such, produce an on-going euphoria. Life is tough, so who wouldn't want this and want to believe it is curing them?

The simple answer is always the best answer. Somehow, somewhere, it was decided that swamping the brain with serotonin would cure depression. A serotonin overload should do it. We fail to recognize that we have such little understanding of the brain to even assume this is true, and you know what they say about assuming. Everyone is then perplexed when they take one brand of antidepressant and then another and another, and they are not cured. In fact, often they get worse, seeing as the side effects are suicidality and depression. So what does the med doctor do when these symptoms appear? They up the dose, of course! So now you are not only more depressed AND suicidal, you are heading into a catatonic stupor and barely able to move, which will prevent you from doing the things that will actually help you recover. Your 15 minutes with the doctor, but more frequently the nurse, as they are more plentiful AND cheaper, is up. Next, please. One of the critical variables to recovery, which is a genuine, caring relationship, goes out the window. There recently was a study at Cambridge University that concluded serotonin has nothing to do with depression. It was a blip on the radar screen and disappeared. Why? Because all the antidepressant drugs rely on giving you serotonin. It speaks to the power of the pharmaceutical industry.

"I can't focus. It is hard for me to concentrate." You must have ADHD. There is no recognition that humans cannot focus for very long to begin with. Remember all diagnoses in the DSM are fabricated, so one fabrication is based on another—fabrication to the second power, so to speak. Recall that being homosexual was once a diagnosis but then vanished from the

DSM. Why? Were all homosexual people "cured"? I suppose not, if it was never a diagnosis in the first place. Poof, be gone!

The most recent proposed "diagnosis" is that of someone not eating a wide enough array of foods. The possibilities are endless with this one. Do we do a study on kids who basically eat macaroni and cheese to see if they are neurotic? This is what all kids do—just eat one or two or maybe three foods of their choice; then all kids are neurotic. This disorder would not have happened back in the day because those kids would still be sitting in front of a plate of green beans until it was eaten.

We live in a culture going at warp speed, AND we are all unique, for better or for worse. We all have the "focusing gene," to whatever degree we have it. That does not make this an illness. If a kid needs more time, a quieter space, someone to read the questions to him, I say just do it.

Ever wonder why most of the students in the classroom with behavioral and "focusing issues" are boys? Compound this with the many living in chaotic homes with parents looking for me time, and it spreads to the girls. Perhaps there is a hormone link? Let's just leave this alone before someone proposes shooting the boys up with female hormones to cure their ADHD. Oh wait, we are already doing this to "straighten out" their sexual identity. The anxiety, depression, and inability to focus caused by this will then be cured, as well as their ADHD and, I am guessing, autism. STOP! If they want hormones as an adult and are fully developed, that is their choice. Injecting children is not a good choice.

This truism that boys are generally more active goes back to the dark ages when I was in grammar school. The "cure" was several recesses during the day. As I had mentioned, Harvard more recently did a study where they let kids run around randomly twice a day. And guess what? They cured all cases of ADHD! What is common sense now has "scientific validity."

But why has this divine revelation not been broadcast? The line of kids snaking around the building getting their meds is part of the reason. As much as the constitution likes to espouse that we are all created equal, this does not mean that we are all created the same. How about we "vive la difference?" Wouldn't that be something? Where hallucinations make someone different, valued just like folks with red hair, for instance. Both are genetic anomalies, so why not? There are cultures where the person having hallucinations is deified. I was not referring to the girls who had visions of the Virgin Mary, but yes, that would fit in nicely.

I knew we were doomed when one of the courses at my alma mater was short-term therapy. There are no shortcuts to developing a real, healthy, and caring relationship. Just ask Sigmund. The short term fits well and supports the drug culture as well as the agenda of the insurance lobbyists. So, what's to lose? Plenty! Your physical and mental health, as well as your life. It is not only the length, but also the quality of the relationship that ultimately will support recovery. As people are unique, the length of time in therapy is unique. Rogers was on target with his "unconditional positive regard." Call it what you like, but this is the nature of the therapeutic relationship and program that is required if folks are to recover, be healed, or be "cured."

The cure is living your life to its fullest. This relationship can happen anywhere but rarely does in our culture. Priests and grandparents used to offer this but rarely do today. People are not flocking to organized religion anymore, particularly after the sex abuse scandal. This type of relationship is critical to "the cure." The "mental health crisis" reflects folks looking for this relationship. Sometimes they find it, but more frequently, they don't.

I have observed that people get into this work for one of three reasons: The courses looked interesting, they genuinely want to help people, or they want the power and control over others. The first two reasons will "do no harm," and the third, of course, will do great harm. As the influence of the church has dwindled, the demand for therapists has increased. Say a few Hail Marys and be on your way. Kind of like short-term therapy. Do a few confessions and be on your way. To wield your authority or power based on a house of straw is an abomination to people coming to you who are struggling and vulnerable. To give some therapists credit, it does take time to figure out that the psychiatric house they work in is made of straw and some never do. "Pay no attention to the man behind the curtain," and some never do. Freud was nominated for the Nobel Prize thirteen times. He was denied thirteen times as his work was "unscientific."

I have witnessed the plethora of dog-and-pony shows over my many years of working in what can be inhuman human services. This applies to the many psychological "tools" that this has produced. Whatever happened to the Stanford-Binet and intelligence testing? Ink blots? And so on. All replaced by the "new and improved" tool for whatever, guaranteed to make big bucks. How about the SATs? Guaranteed to make big bucks, but not guaranteed to reveal who are the "best and the brightest."

Currently, we have CBT, DBT, CVS (just added the last one to see if you were paying attention), and, more recently, "trauma therapy," with unlimited variations on this theme. Perfect. None of us get out of this thing we call life without trauma. This has led to folks being "traumatized" by things like parents having to work and being "abandoned" in after-school care. I think it would be far more traumatic if they didn't work and were without food and shelter. Yes, people do have trauma that is truly heartbreaking, but we have turned what is normal trauma into an illness, just as everything else in the DSM. Trauma is the current dog and pony show. Desertion by parents, drug abuse, random acts of nature and humans, car accidents, sexual abuse. The list of actual trauma is long, but when people come to us for help, we do them no favor by having trauma dictate their destiny.

I sat one day with the poor woman trying to supervise me. God help her for this and for what I could see her actual job was. It was taking call after call from folks looking for psychiatric drugs. The popular ones like Klonopin, Gabapentin, and Adderall make life a bit more bearable, but at what price? All of the drugs that allow you to face life pleasantly sedated or hyped up come at a price. If you have the predisposition towards addiction, these drugs will surely kick it off. How ironic. You go seeking medical care and end up in worse condition than when you started. "Do no harm!" Trauma is part of the life process.

The mental health clinic on the college campus has become the candy store. It's no longer necessary to hit the street to find a thrill. How convenient, how profitable, and how disgusting. The clinic is the place where any student can walk in, and if they know the magic words—and they all do, like "I cannot focus," they will be instantaneously rewarded with a script for Adderall. They can share it with friends, party on (mixing it with alcohol, which is death defying), sell it, or do whatever fits their whim at the moment. Adderall is an opportunity not to improve your study habits but to party on and then use it to stay up all night before an exam. And I had to use 10 pots of coffee. How far we have come!

Let me tell you a story about a kid who received Adderall this way. In the interest of anonymity, I will use ALL pronouns, he/she/they, although "they" still perplexes me. Unfortunately, he/she/they had the genetic make up that predisposed "them" towards addiction. Not that we know much about this either, but the kid's dad had an addiction that ruined what began as a very promising life. He/she/they originally took the drug as prescribed, and then he/she/they did not. The drug came within a hair of killing him/her/them. The grace of God saved he/she/they.

The story gets better and makes a wonderful point about the mental health/psychiatric system. I think I'll call him/her/they a he/him in the interest of brevity. I hate typing, and all of those pronouns are wearing me out. He went into therapy. The "prescriber," as the drug dispensers in psychiatry are called, since this is all they do, was informed of the addiction by a licensed, qualified therapist in the field. (As an aside, licensing is a relatively new phenomenon being dictated by the insurance companies and in no way assures you of a competent therapist/provider.) The prescriber agreed, to be certain, that there would be NO MORE Adderall prescribed. Lo and behold, a couple of months later, the kid had his Adderall prescription back! It nearly killed him, and the prescribee, or unsuspecting victim, won a lawsuit against the prescriber.

How do you put a value on almost totally ruining a young life full of potential and nearly killing him? The monetary settlement reflects our values as a culture that somehow the "damage done" can be rectified this way. Behold the malpractice lawyers who can afford a cottage at Little Compton. Behold the human service worker who can barely pay their rent. Personally, I'd rather see the prescriber take his drugs in massive quantities involuntarily, as this is what addiction amounts to.

So, Adderall is off limits, maybe and maybe not. Adderall has now been replaced with "nonaddictive" gabapentin, which we all know is highly addictive. This is the ongoing ruse that the pharmaceutical companies dupe the doctors with. Some of whom care about this, and many do not. Think opioid crisis.

Initially, the addictive potential was not recognized and/or glossed over, no big deal. Why? Big money. The other reason this is so easy to do is that we have little hard data, scientific proof, as to why one person gets addicted and not the next. There are many theories and observations, just like in the rest of the field of psychology, and the many dog-and-pony shows. If we actually knew, we could cure addiction, which as AA has espoused for many decades, we cannot.

So what is the "cure" for mental health problems? For some, the symptoms can go away, and we truthfully don't know why. And for others, the symptoms remain, yet they live fulfilling lives in spite of this.

You might ask, what is the answer, dear psychological guru? As the good witch once said to Dorothy, "It was there all the time," and Dorothy then tapped the heels of the ruby slippers three times. Shall we start with the current drug-dealing being done by psychiatry and more recently by nurse practitioners who are cheaper to employ? There was a time when only MDs could prescribe. This power has now been opened up to nurses. Why? Well, they are not as cheap as say social workers, but they are much cheaper than MDs, and this fits so nicely for the insurance companies. There also is a shortage of psychiatrists. Who would want to spend a lifetime in school and then be relegated to writing scripts that might be effective and generally are not? Your 15 minutes are up. Even Freud, the "father of psychiatry," based his work on long-term relationships.

Let me outline the typical mental "health" scenario. The patient comes in and says, "I am depressed." The patient gets labeled with an arbitrary diagnosis from the DSM, per regulations of the insurance companies. No money, no therapy. Then, the patient "complies" with "therapy," to no avail. The dosage is upped, of course. When this doesn't work, a slew of other drugs will be tried, and the greater percentage fail. There is always the placebo effect. The patient hits the psychiatric jackpot and is "cured" thanks to the miracle of drugs. Not really. If you get the right drug and walk around slightly but pleasantly high all the time, doesn't this beat reality?

Then try to get off these "nonaddictive" and "harmless" drugs. If you quit cold turkey, you could end up a dead turkey or quivering in the corner from the effects of withdrawal from these "nonaddictive" substances. Aha! I quit taking the drug, and my depression, ADHD, anxiety, and whatever symptoms returned. No, you are in withdrawal. Believe what you choose. Often, someone who states they are depressed becomes suicidal after taking the antidepressants. Why, oh why? As "they" say, it doesn't take a rocket scientist to figure it out. Just read the side effects.

The anti-anxiety drugs do help many and generally will lose their effectiveness over time. We have discussed Adderall. If your body is going at warp speed, you can deduce what the harm will be, including addiction. Adderall used to be called "bennies," "uppers"; it's the same deal. Pass at your own risk. Not to mention, a generation of kids have been given these drugs with abandon. Let me know in about 20 years how that works out. The recent finding that increased serotonin does not "cure" depression appears to have been repressed. This is the cornerstone of ALL the antidepressants. Is it a wonder that most folks find these drugs ineffective?

I can continue but don't want to bore you, so I will get to the point. A friend of mine just said she has read how microdoses of LSD will "cure" mental illness. Haven't we been here before? Micro, macro doses, supervised, unsupervised. There will always be folks who feel they are "cured" from whatever new/old dog-and-pony show comes to the fore. Give me hard scientific data, not some freewheeling hypothesis. This too shall pass, with all of the resulting train wrecks in its path. It is a very substantial risk to take for anyone already feeling they are struggling with their sanity.

So what does work? Anyone who has experienced an actual clubhouse model will attest to what I am saying. This clubhouse effect can be repeated in individual psychotherapy but at a high cost to the therapist and "therapee." You are having one person do the work of what requires a village. Perhaps there are other villages somewhere, but at this point, I have not seen them. I am not speaking of a clubhouse knock-off usually under the direction of a mental health center, but an actual living, breathing, affirming, unconditionally loving clubhouse. It is magic.

Some of those who have been "institutionalized" by the current mental health system (i.e., clinics) may never be able to fully benefit. "Institutionalization" is not done just in the state hospitals; we have transferred it to the community. Many have been turned into professional patients who are compliant with their med regimes and compliant with the debilitating messages being given to them through day programs, individual "therapy," and group "therapy" run by the mental health centers.

I often wonder if the director where I formerly worked is worried that if folks actually recover, she will run out of paying customers. Customers who support her and other administrators' excessive salaries. This is not Amazon, and the money was to go into programs and not into their pockets. Unfortunately, until there are major cultural changes, there will be plenty of customers.

The original model, Fountain House, is in NYC on the edge of Hell's Kitchen. The program is located in a beautiful old brownstone, complete with oriental rugs and chandeliers. The founders and cornerstone were two moms whose children had been institutionalized. After "deinstitutionalization," their kids were spending their time sitting on the steps of the NYC public library. We delude ourselves that we are far more humane by having the community mental health centers run the services just like the state hospital but located in the community. Does it really matter where the state hospital is located? It is the same institution where people become institutionalized.

The underpinnings of any approach that will find success and "cure" folks is an approach that is based on GENUINE caring and concern. Compassion and hope for a better future. You can dress it up however you like: cognitive, behavioral, whatever. But when anyone recovers, this is what is underneath and the theme you will hear in the background. A program located in a garage complete with fumes, or in a clinic with separate but equal entrances for staff and clients, does not give the message of being cared about and the hope that those moms projected. It is the physical, emotional, and spiritual environment that heals.

The relationships in the clubhouse can be mirrored by therapists promoting compassion, understanding, growth, recovery, and hope. This will be condemned as violating "policy," crossing professional boundaries, causing insurance liability, and so on. Please note that professional ethics still stand. There is no dating or putting anyone in a subservient role. One of the most eye-opening moments for me was when I realized that "staff meetings" at the club and elsewhere pretty much were a place to vent and create walls between staff and clients. Tear down those walls, and you will reveal an entire social system happening outside your purview. If we are not totally honest, there is no "cure." In the clinic and mental health centers, there is no we; there is us and them.

As I had mentioned, people choosing to work in human services can be put into one of three categories: those who truly care and want to change the world, those who revel in and abuse the power they have over folks when they are vulnerable, and those who couldn't figure out what they wanted to do and the psychology courses looked interesting. If you fall into the latter two categories, please change your profession immediately. "Do no harm." Whatever work we must do it must be under the leadership of those who truly care.

So, what is the reality? Well, moms being moms, they wanted more for their kids than hanging out in the brownstone. They wanted more than "day treatment"—programs and crocheting groups. This is not easy work for those supporting and those being supported. I wore out many pairs of high heels going from one place to the next, looking for jobs in all the wrong places. They did not want to hire "those people" unless, of course, one of them happened to be someone they loved.

The way to solve the mass shootings is "more mental health services." Yes, more quality services are sorely needed, not more of what we currently have. However, mental illness is NOT the cause of mass shootings. Folks labeled "mentally ill" are no more likely to be violent than "normal" people, whatever that means. How often do you hear that it was "such a shock; we never would have expected he would have done that"? Or the opposite: "Yeah, it was to be expected; he has a history of mental illness"? Neither statement has anything to do with the real causes.

The "services" (call them what you wish) at Fountain House grew out of the needs, desires, and dreams of those who loved them. At Genesis, we planned these services together—not in an "ivory tower," thinking that the world would conform to our ideas. It amazed me how few of my cohorts had actual, substantial experience in the work we supposedly were preparing folks to do when I taught at the college level. This partially explains why the newly minted student comes with the delusion that memorizing so-and-so's approach will lead to curing everyone who comes to us. This or that approach provides the keys to the castle, if only you can master it properly. This is a total illusion, of course.

The formula is simple. What does the person want to accomplish, and how do we develop a truly caring relationship and support to do so? For years in the mental health world, a high school diploma was the gold standard, and all were happy with this. Just like all were happy spending their days in a sheltered workshop assembling widgets or in the state hospital. Folks wanted more, and the people who loved them wanted more for them.

The community of support that is currently called a clubhouse, in its true form, will invite, welcome, and support recovery. Beware of knock-offs, or those who are a club in name only. So what is an individual therapist to do when this is not available or not being done properly? You find yourself alone. I have been living this for the past 20-plus years. It is not easy nor desirable and may not allow for as much potential, but it is possible. Some are so turned off by "programs" and "groups" that your support initially is all there is. So just do it. Look for jobs, housing, friends, and meaning in life together. Give folks your personal cell number; it will not be abused and gives comfort with little effort. Once the process of recovery kicks in, you and he/she may be amazed. A real club is open 365 days a year, and initially, people will go there as they need to and choose to. Attendance will taper off as they have their own life and live it. The exception, of course, is those who chose the club as their career. How simple.

I hope you now understand what "the cure" is. Perhaps someday, there will be better answers, but what is better than having a relationship with someone who truly cares for your well-being? I suppose the answer is having a community that truly cares and will be there for you for life. Sort of like your mom and a good marriage. Except unlike the marriage, you can come and go as you please.

The answer will not be in pill form, although that is what we demand in our culture. There will be no total answer in all the dog-and-pony show facilitators seeking their 15 minutes of fame and quick money. The key will be in your dedication, compassion, caring, belief in equality, and love of the work and the "clients." This cannot be taught. I know caring when I see it. I know control when I see it, and so do you. As the expression goes, "Walk beside them, not in front or behind." Simple, yes. Easy, no.

Parting Words

Acknowledgments

Thank you to my family for your many forms of support. To Marguerite, my very smart and beautiful daughter. Thank you for your medical expertise and being my best buddy.

To Douglas, thank you for all you do, outside of the medical issues of course.

Thank you to cousin Deb, my first best buddy and still my very special friend. Your honesty and love are amazing in a sea of family issues, shall we say.

To Suzanne and Jim my adopted family, who came to my rescue yet again when we were homeless yet again....

And Dinnis, you have always been family as you have always been there for me. You always seemed to notice the little things like when we had no heat.

Tam who we love and had it not been for her would not have found David.

Thank you, David, for your kindness and support through this book journey and understanding the things that have delayed the process.

Thank you, Jack, from Fountainhouse whose support and kindness helped us remember the ideals and values that work.

To Renee and Joel despite what looked like overwhelming responsibilities you found a place in your schedule and in your heart to try and give the folks in Athol Ma a decent place to go.

Millie, you were amazing and I am honored to have called you friend. You taught me lessons about life, mental health and friendship that are invaluable and never taught in school.

Adriana, the path you chose was very, very difficult. Your strength and you are so admirable.

And Kim, you have a beautiful heart and I know you are also strong and talented.

Heather your realness and humor are always a pleasure.

Andre, my hope is for you to win this battle, keep on fighting,

Thank you, Nancy, for your wisdom, kindness and support. It's wonderful to know there are a few of us left.

Ronnie, your warm welcome and friendship are truly treasured and I reflect on how fortunate I am to have such a lovely friend and neighbor, thank you.

To Jacob, your humor, strength, and loving nature are welcome additions to this world we live in.

Jane and Charlie, you are two of the most amazing people I am honored to call friend, thank you.

Thank you Christian for your help and support, I am grateful that you opened your heart to a cause that means much to me and many.

Appendix:

Where to Read, Watch, and Learn about All Things Mental Health

Dear Friend, from My Life I Write to You in Your Life, Yiyun Li – Deals with recovery from suicidal urges

The Future of the Mind: The Scientific Quest to Understand, Enhance, and Empower the Mind, Michio Kaku – Reveals how little actual science we have about the mind/brain

The Myth of Mental Illness: Foundations of a Theory of Personal Conduct, Thomas S. Szasz – This was the classic expose of it's time. Still relevant.

One Flew Over the Cuckoo's Nest, Ken Kesey – A classic and an expose. The problems in the "asylums" did not disappear. They were simply moved to the community. And much remains the same…

About the Author

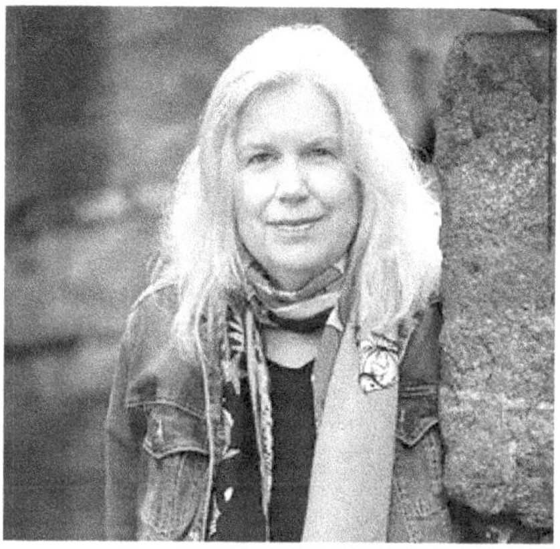

I was dead and wrote four books.

And no, I am not a zombie.

During a hospital visit, I was given an antibiotic that I was allergic to and ended up on life support with a 2% chance to live. While I was in the coma, I travelled to the netherworld and visited my dad, mom and grandmother who had all passed. I remember in the middle of our conversation; my dad suddenly turned and told me to leave as quickly as possible. I remember running and became very short of breath. My children instantly appeared in front of me. I grabbed them and hugged them with all my might. Then, everything vanished.

A nurse looked down at me and smiled and said, "Welcome back."

My first thought was welcome back to where? When I came to my senses, my thoughts turned to the meaning of my experience. It became obvious that I returned to care for my children. However, there was a nagging sense of urgency that remained with me. What was it? This haunted me.

The doctor had forbidden me to return to my job at that time working as a psychotherapist with single moms. In response, I began writing a book about single parenting in a multiracial and multigenerational setting in my myopic condition. I may be a mess but my brain still worked! I figured I could still provide comfort to single moms even if I could not meet with them at the time.

I kept thinking back to my visit with my dad and reflecting on the meaning of it. I realized that I had to write his story because when I die his story will die with me. He was a social and political activist and ran for president numerous times. He tread on the toes of the big boys of his era, ex-president Richard Nixon and Nelson Rockefeller. This highly decorated WWII veteran was driven by them out of the country. My nearsightedness did not allow me to see what was a common thread to what was now two books.

Onward. The next book was also a social mission. It is a work in progress tentatively titled "The Cure for Mental Illness." My life long dedication to teaching, starting innovative programs and psychotherapy lead to a pressing concern about the quality of mental health services. I needed to get the truth out so the mental health system would "do no harm."

The next book came alive when I did a few sketches to entertain a friend's severely autistic daughter. Because she loved Mr. Muffinstuff (my adored shih tzu), it was only appropriate that he have a book of his own. Mr. Muffinstuff began his life as a lost puppy. I came to realize that his story was also the story of many of the kids I had worked with. The book is the story of Mr. Muffinstuff's trauma and ends with a happily ever after. The book aims to relay a message of hope for these kids.

After drafting these books, the mission was clear to me. I often tell my folks in therapy I wish I had a magic wand to fix "it." It became clear that I do have a wand to fix "it." The wand is to share a lifetime of my personal and professional challenges and victories to help the folks looking for hope.

Nobody lives long enough to make the changes needed in this world. Perhaps this is by design, but we can at least pass on the knowledge of a lifetime. This was the reason I had a death experience and returned. The time for me to do this is now because my next death experience will not include a return ticket.

www.ingramcontent.com/pod-product-compliance
Lightning Source LLC
LaVergne TN
LVHW022312200926
848481LV00004B/1304
9798893900040